# COOKBOOK
# FOR
# BEGINNERS

*Very Easy and Delicious Recipes to Get you Started in the Kitchen*

**Gillian Tambor**

no scenarios in which the publisher or the original author of this work can be in any fashion deemed liable for any hardship or damages that may befall them after undertaking information described herein.

Additionally, the information in the following pages is intended only for informational purposes and should thus be thought of as universal. As befitting its nature, it is presented without assurance regarding its prolonged validity or interim quality. Trademarks that are mentioned are done without written consent and can in no way be considered an endorsement from the trademark holder.

# TABLE OF CONTENTS

# Introduction

Would you like to learn how to cook?

However, does this seem like something impossible to you?

Eating is fun, just like preparing it if you do it right.

Because food preparation is not mathematical science and if you cook something yourself, it tastes even better.

Anyone can learn to cook, but it is important to have a little patience at the beginning and start with simple dishes. After gaining enough experience you will also be able to prepare more complicated recipes.

Surely it is easier and faster to book your dinner or lunch at a restaurant or home delivery.

But cooking alone has decisive notices. One of them is that cooking can relax and reduce stress. This is why many see cooking as a meditative activity.

Another benefit is that when you cook on your own, you tend to eat healthier foods. Because fresh ingredients are mostly used in cooking, means you consume a host of valuable nutrients - nutrients that are usually lacking in pizzas or frozen snacks around the corner. So, cooking yourself has positive effects on your health and you will soon feel more vital. Another advantage is the noteworthy economic savings.

For example, it's cheaper to buy lettuce, cucumber, and tomatoes individually first than to grab a salad from the refrigerated counter. The same goes for most dishes that can be bought as ready-made products.

However, beginners in particular often make mistakes that put a damper on their pleasure in cooking and can be easily avoided.

Be patient, because progress comes step by step and you will surely notice that the more often you prepare a dish, the better it will be. This includes ensuring that you don't approach the matter with too high expectations of your cooking skills. Because especially at the beginning you make one or two mistakes when cooking, which is why the dish does not always turn out perfectly.

Another common mistake is that novice cooks are not familiar with their kitchen. On the one hand, this means that you should check that you have all the necessary kitchen appliances. After all, it would be annoying if you noticed in the middle of the preparation that you have neither a mixer nor a hand blender, but now you have to puree something. You should also know how long it takes your oven to heat up and how quickly your stove can bring water to a boil. This allows you to plan the individual steps better and to proceed more efficiently.

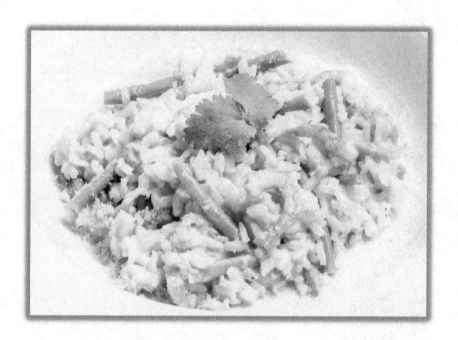

# Recipes

# Avocado French Toast

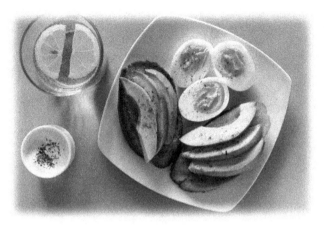

Time required:
35 minutes

Servings: 02

## INGREDIENTS

*1 avocado*
*3 eggs*
*4 teaspoons of
tomato pesto*
*4 slices of sandwich
toast*
*150 ml milk*
*1 pinch of chili flakes*
*2 tbsp clarified
butter*
*2 teaspoons of
lemon juice salt*

## STEPS FOR COOKING

1. Cut the avocado in half, core and remove the peel. Put the pulp in a bowl and use a fork to crush the pulp as fine as possible. Then mix with salt, chili flakes and lemon juice.

2. Whisk the milk and eggs in a casserole dish and season with salt.

3. Brush 2 of the toast slices with 2 teaspoons of tomato pesto each and then with the avocado cream. Now place one of the remaining two toast slices on top.

4. Now put the sandwiches in the baking dish with the egg cream. Let it steep for 3-4 minutes, then turn over and let it steep for another 3-4 minutes on the other side. The egg cream should be completely absorbed by the toast.

| INGREDIENTS | STEPS FOR COOKING |
|---|---|

5. Heat a coated pan and add the clarified butter. Now put the two sandwiches in the pan and fry each side for about 5 minutes over medium heat until they are light brown.

6. Remove and drain on kitchen paper. Then serve immediately.

# Easy Mozzarella & Pesto Chicken Casserole

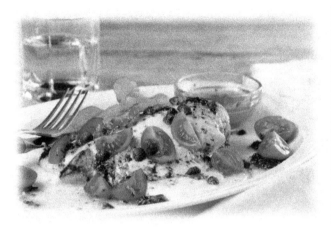

Time required:
60 minutes

Servings: 04

## INGREDIENTS

¼ cup pesto,

8 oz. cream cheese softened

¼ - ½ - cup heavy cream

8 oz. mozzarella cubed

2 lb. cooked cubed chicken breasts

8 oz. mozzarella shredded

## STEPS FOR COOKING

1. Preheat stove to 400. Sprinkle a tremendous supper dish with a cooking shower.

2. Unite the underlying three fixings and mix them until smooth in a bread bowl.

3. Incorporate the chicken and cubed mozzarella. Trade to the goulash dish.

4. Sprinkle the decimated mozzarella to complete the process of everything.

5. Plan for 25-30 minutes. Present with zoodles, spinach, or squashed cauliflower.

# Cream Cheese Spinach Omelette

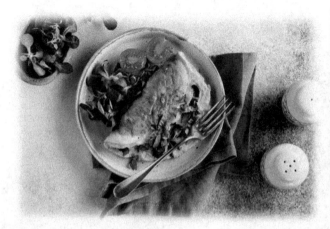

Time required:
15 minutes

Servings: 01

## INGREDIENTS

*2 oz. Cream cheese*

*¼ cup Chopped fresh spinach leaves Large*

*2 eggs*

*¼ teaspoon Toasted sesame seed oil*

## STEPS FOR COOKING

1. Mix cream cheese and spinach, then set aside.

2. Beat two eggs in a separate bowl and set aside as well.

3. Use toasted sesame seed oil and lightly grease the frying pan.

4. Preheat the pan over medium heat, and then pour in the eggs.

5. Cook eggs for 1 minute, then flip it on the other side.

6. Spread cream cheese mixture onto the cooked side of the egg.

7. Fold egg in half. Wait at least 1 minute for the cream cheese mixture to melt.

8. Remove from heat and serve immediately.

# Baked Corned Beef Omelette

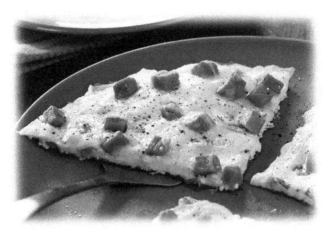

Time required:
55 minutes

Servings: 02

## INGREDIENTS

*2 Large eggs*

*3 ounce Thinly sliced corned beef*

*1 cup Heavy cream*

*1 cup Grated mozzarella cheese*

*1 tbsp.Chopped green onion*

*½ teaspoon Lawry's Seasoned salt*

## STEPS FOR COOKING

1. Preheat oven to 325 degrees.
2. Mix cream, beaten eggs and seasoned salt together.
3. Tear the sliced corned beef into smaller pieces.
4. Add corned beef, cheese, and onion into the egg mixture.
5. Pour the mixture into a greased baking dish.
6. Bake without cover for 45 minutes or until the top is golden brown.

# Low Carb Waffles

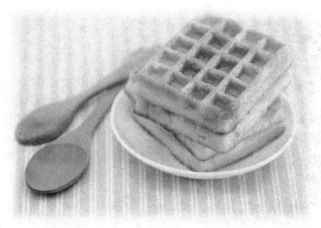

Time required:
35 minutes

Servings: 01

## INGREDIENTS

*3 egg whites*

*2 tablespoons unsweetened almond milk*

*2 tablespoons coconut flour*

*½ teaspoon baking powder Sweetener, optional*

## STEPS FOR COOKING

1. Whip 2 of the egg whites using a hand mixer or egg beater.

2. Stir in the coconut flour, milk, baking powder, sweetener, and 1 egg white.

3. Heat up the waffle iron and grease with a nonstick spray.

4. Pour in the batter and cook in the waffle iron for 3 to 4 minutes until browned.

5. Pull it out and serve. Enjoy.

# Banana Porridge

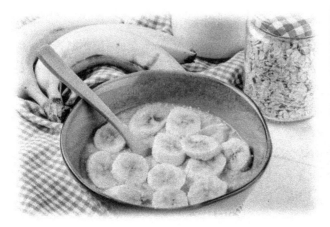

Time required:
15 minutes

Servings: 04

## INGREDIENTS

2 ripe bananas,
peeled and mashed
¾ cup almond meal
¼ cup flax meal
½ teaspoon ground
ginger
1 teaspoon ground
cinnamon
1/8 teaspoon
ground nutmeg
1/8 teaspoon
ground cloves
Salt, to taste
2 cups coconut milk

## STEPS FOR COOKING

1. In a pan, mix together all ingredients on medium-low heat.
2. Bring to some gentle simmer, stirring continuously.
3. Cook, stirring continuously for approximately 2-3 minutes or till desired consis10cy.
4. Serve using your desired topping.

# Eggs in Avocado Cup

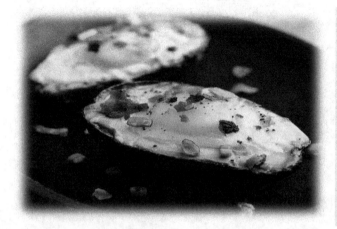

Time required:
10 minutes

Servings: 02

## INGREDIENTS

2 ripe avocados,
halved, pitted and
scooped out about 2
tablespoons of flesh
4 organic eggs
Salt and freshly
ground black
pepper, to taste
1 tablespoon chives,
minced

## STEPS FOR COOKING

1. Preheat the oven to 425 degrees F.
2. Arrange the avocado halves in a small baking dish.
3. In a smaller, bowl, break an egg after which carefully transfer into within an avocado half.
4. Repeat with remaining eggs.
5. Bake approximately 15-twenty minutes or till desired doneness.
6. Serve immediately with all the sprinkling of salt, black pepper and chives.

# Apple Omelet

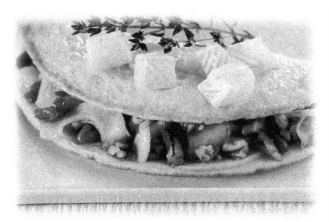

Time required:
15 minutes

Servings: 01

## INGREDIENTS

*2 teaspoons coconut oil, divided*

*½ of enormous green apple, cored and sliced thinly*

*¼ teaspoon ground cinnamon*

*1/8 teaspoon ground nutmeg*

*2 large organic eggs*

*1/8 teaspoon organic vanilla extract*

*Pinch of salt*

*Maple syrup, if desired*

## STEPS FOR COOKING

1. In a nonstick frying pan, heat 1 teaspoon of oil on medium- low heat.

2. Add apple slices and sprinkle with nutmeg and cinnamon.

3. Cook for approximately 4-5 minutes, turning once inside middle.

4. Meanwhile inside a bowl, add eggs, vanilla and salt and beat till fluffy.

5. Add remaining oil inside the pan and let it melt completely.

6. Place the egg mixture over apple slices evenly.

7. Cook for approximately 3-4 minutes or till desired doneness.

8. Carefully, turn the pan over a serving plate and immediately, fold the omelet.

# Creamy Avocado Soup

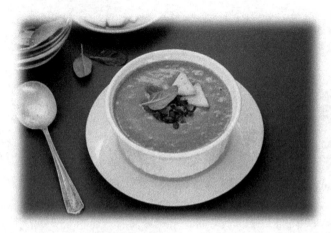

Time required:
20 minutes

Servings: 06

## INGREDIENTS

2 avocados, peel and pitted

2 cups vegetable stock

1 tbsp. fresh lemon juice

3/4 cup heavy cream

2 tbsp. dry sherry

Pepper

Salt

## STEPS FOR COOKING

1. Add avocado, lemon juice, sherry, and stock to the blender and blend until smooth.

2. Pour blended mixture into a bowl.

3. Add cream and stir well. Season with pepper and salt. Serve and enjoy.

# Citrus Salmon

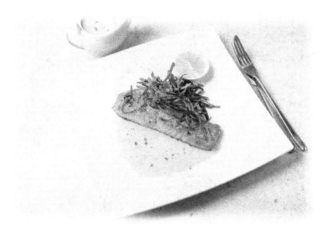

Time required:
45 minutes

Servings: 06

## INGREDIENTS

*2 (1-pound) salmon fillets*

*Salt and ground black pepper, as required 1 tablespoon seafood seasoning*

*2 lemons, sliced*

*2 limes, sliced*

## STEPS FOR COOKING

1. Preheat the "Wood Pellet Smoker and Grill" on a grill set to 225 degrees F.

2. Season the salmon fillets with salt, black pepper, and seafood seasoning evenly.

3. Place the salmon fillets onto the grill and top each with lemon and lime slices evenly.

4. Cook for about half-hour.

5. Remove the salmon fillets from the grill and serve hot.

6. Grill trout for 5 minutes from both sides (be careful not to overcook the fish).

7. Pour fish with marinade and serve hot with lemon slices.

# Spaghetti Squash Casserole

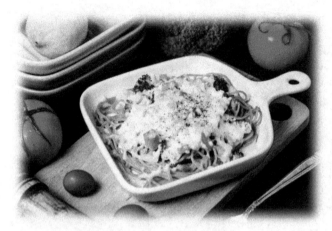

Time required:
45 minutes

Servings: 06

## INGREDIENTS

*1 spaghetti squash cooked*

*1 pound lean ground beef*

*1 onion diced*

*2 cloves garlic minced*

*15 ounces diced tomatoes canned*

*1 tablespoon tomato paste*

*1 cup marinara sauce or pasta sauce*

*1 teaspoon Italian seasoning*

*1 ½ cups mozzarella cheese shredded*

## STEPS FOR COOKING

1. Preheat oven to 375F.
2. Cook squash until tender. Cut in half. Using a fork, remove spaghetti squash strands from the squash and set them aside.
3. In a medium saucepan, cook ground beef, onion, and garlic until no pink remains. Drain any fat.
4. Add diced tomatoes, tomato paste, pasta sauce, and seasoning. Simmer 5 minutes.
5. Stir in squash. Place in a casserole dish (or back into the squash halves) and top with cheese. Bake for 20 minutes or until golden and bubbly.

# Fried Cabbage with Sausage

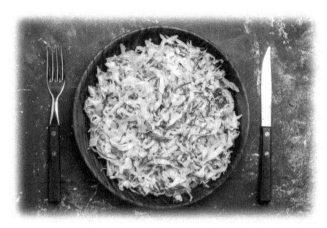

Time required:
35 minutes

Servings: 02

## INGREDIENTS

12 ounces smoked
sausage

2 tablespoons olive
oil divided

1/2 yellow onion

2 cloves garlic

1 medium head
cabbage

1 teaspoon salt

1 teaspoon ground
pepper

## STEPS FOR COOKING

1. Slice the smoked sausage into thin rounds.

2. Heat 1 tablespoon olive oil in a dutch oven or large, deep skillet over medium heat. Add the sausage to the skillet and cook, stirring often, until sausage is browned on both sides, about 4 minutes.

3. Add the onion and garlic to the skillet and cook for 3 more minutes to soften onions.

4. Add the remaining tablespoon of oil to the skillet along with the cabbage and sprinkle with salt and pepper.

5. Cook the cabbage, stirring constantly, until it becomes tender, about 10 minutes.

6. Serve immediately.

# Beef and Broccoli Stir Fry

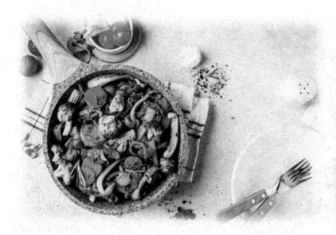

Time required:
25 minutes

Servings: 02

## INGREDIENTS

2½ Tbsp, divided cornstarch

¼ tsp Table salt

¾ pound(s), thinly sliced against the grain Uncooked lean trimmed sirloin beef

2 tsp Canola oil

1 cup of(s), divided chicken broth

cup of(s), florets (about a 12 oz bag), Uncooked broccoli

1 Tbsp, fresh, minced Ginger root

2 tsp minced garlic

¼ tsp, or as need Red pepper flakes

## STEPS FOR COOKING

1. Toss the beef with 2 tablespoons, cornstarch, and salt on a pan.

2. Over medium-high flame, heat the oil in a big nonstick wok or deep skillet. Stir-fry the beef for 4 minutes, or until it is finely browned and cooked through; move to a bowl with a slotted spoon.

3. In the same skillet, add 1/2 cup broth and stir to loosen some stuck-on food. Cook until broccoli is almost crisp-tender, around 3 minutes, flipping regularly and sprinkling with a tablespoon of water if required. Uncover the pan and stir-fry the ginger, garlic, and red pepper flakes for around 1 minute, or until fragrant.

4. Stir together the remaining 1/2 cup broth, water, soy sauce, and 1/2 tbsp

*¼ cup of Water*

*¼ cup of soy sauce*

cornstarch in a cup until smooth; pour into the pan. Reduce heat to medium-low and bring to a simmer; cook, occasionally stirring, for 1 minute or until slightly thickened.

5. Return the beef to the plate, along with any remaining juices, and toss to combine. Assist per serving, approximately 1 1/4 cup.

# Salmon Burgers with Lemon Butter and Mash

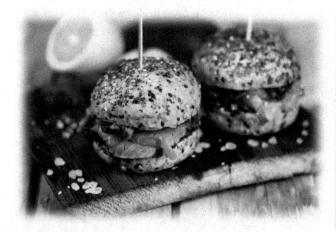

Time required:
70 minutes

Servings: 04

## INGREDIENTS

**For the Salmon Burgers:**
2 pounds salmon
One egg
1/2 yellow onion
1 tsp. salt
1/2 tsp. black pepper
2 ounces butter
**For the Green Mash:**
1-pound broccoli
5 ounces of butter
2 ounces parmesan cheese
Pepper

## STEPS FOR COOKING

1. Warm-up your oven at 100 degrees.
2. Cut the salmon into small pieces. Combine all the burger items with the fish in a blender. Pulse for thirty seconds. Make eight patties.
3. Warm-up butter in an iron skillet. Fry the burgers for five minutes.
4. Boil water, along with some salt in a pot, put the broccoli florets. Cook for three to four minutes. Drain. Add parmesan cheese and butter. Blend the ingredients using an immersion blender. Add pepper and salt.
5. Combine lemon juice with butter, pepper, and salt. Beat using an electric beater.

## INGREDIENTS

salt

**For the Lemon Butter:**

4 ounces butter

2 tbsps. lemon juice

Pepper

salt

## STEPS FOR COOKING

6. Put a dollop of lemon butter on the top and green mash by the side. Serve.

# Smoked and Hearty Cabbage

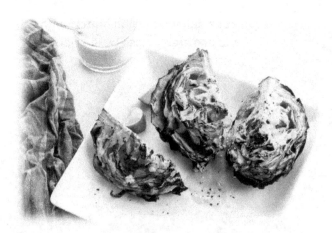

Time required:
35 minutes

Servings: 04

## INGREDIENTS

8 ounces smoked fish (trout, salmon, sturgeon or sable), bones removed and broken into small pieces

½ head cabbage

4 tablespoons unsalted butter

½ cup heavy cream

½ lemon, sliced thinly

1 teaspoon lemon zest

½ teaspoon black pepper

2 tablespoons fresh parsley

## STEPS FOR COOKING

1. Boil salted water in a pot. Quarter cabbage and cut into ½ strips.

2. Cook cabbage for a few minutes.

3. Melt 2 tablespoons butter in a pan over medium heat.

4. Put the cabbage. Cook and stir gently. Pour cream.

5. Put a dash of pepper and add the lemon rind.

6. Cook for 5 minutes. Place the smoked fish in the skillet. Cook for 3 minutes.

7. The other remaining 2 tablespoons of butter melt it in a cup.

8. Drizzle over fish. Garnish with lemon slices and parsley. Serve and enjoy.

# Italian Poached Eggs

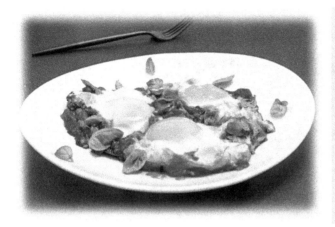

Time required:
15 minutes

Servings: 02

## INGREDIENTS

*16 oz Marinara Sauce lowest sugar available*

*3-4 pieces jarred roasted red pepper, sliced eggs*

*Pinch every salt and pepper*

*leaves fresh basil, torn into small pieces*

## STEPS FOR COOKING

1. Preheat a deep-rimmed skillet over high heat.
2. Add marinara sauce and sliced red peppers.
3. Build a "well" with the back of a spoon and crack one egg into it. Rep with the remaining three eggs.
4. Season to taste with salt and pepper.
5. Allow for about 12 minutes of cooking time or until the eggs are firm when shaken in the pan. (For the last 2 minutes, I covered it with a lid.)
6. Remove from heat, sprinkle with torn basil and scoop onto plate or bowl.

# Easy Fish Tacos

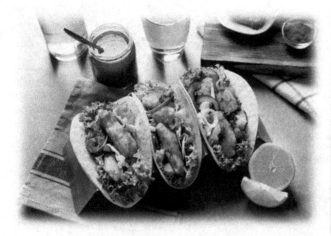

Time required:
20 minutes

Servings: 02

## INGREDIENTS

¼ cup cottage cheese

¼ cup yogurt

¼ tsp cumin seeds

half of a lime Juice

2 cups shredded cabbage

1 chopped tomato

**For Tacos:**

1 pound raw shrimp, shelled and deveined, tails removed

1 tsp olive oil

½ tsp cumin seeds

Cilantro (garnish)

Chopped Green onion

## STEPS FOR COOKING

1. Combine cottage cheese, yogurt, cumin, salt, and lime juice in a mixing bowl. Toss in the cabbage and tomato. Combine all ingredients and set aside.

2. Combine the shrimp, olive oil, and cumin in a mixing bowl. 5-10 minutes over medium heat, sauté the shrimp mixture in a saucepan (until shrimp are cooked through). Remove the pan from the sun.

3. If you're going to eat the tortillas, heat them first. Then cover with the fried shrimp mixture. After that, top with the sauce mixture and cilantro, and green onions.

## INGREDIENTS

*(garnish)Chopped*
*Corn tortilla*

## STEPS FOR COOKING

# Broiled Tilapia with Parmesan Cheese

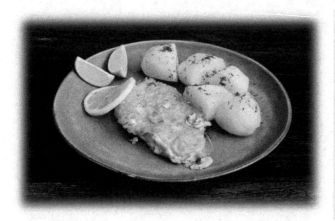

Time required:
15 minutes

Servings: 02

## INGREDIENTS

*(4) 4 oz Tilapia fillets*

*2 tablespoon grated parmesan cheese*

*1 tablespoon light mayonnaise*

*1 tablespoon lime juice*

*1 teaspoon garlic chopped*

*1/2 teaspoon dill weed dried Sea salt*

## STEPS FOR COOKING

1. Place the tilapia fillets on a broiling pan, sprinkle with 1/2 of the dill weed and a pinch of salt, and broil for 2-3 minutes on the top rack of the oven. While the fish is broiling, combine the remaining ingredients, including the remaining dill.

2. Take out the tilapia from the oven and spread the parmesan mixture on top.

3. Then, take the fish to the oven for a second or two under the broiler.

4. If you're using frozen Tilapia filets, bake them according to the package instructions first, then top with the coating and broil. Alternatively, you should coat the fish and bake it according to the package instructions.

5. At this point in the diet, asparagus may not be suitable.

# Garden Fresh Salad

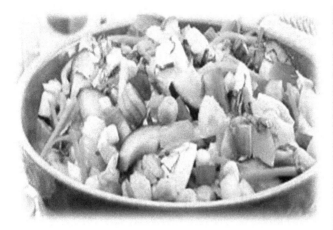

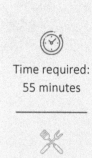

Time required:
55 minutes

Servings: 02

## INGREDIENTS

*2 tbsp butter*

*1½ cup broccoli, cut into flowerets*

*1½ cup spring onion, cut into small pieces / diced*

*1 cup green pepper, cut into small cubes*

*½ cup tomato, cut into small cubes*

*1 small onion, cut into small pieces*

*½ teaspoon black pepper powder*

*Salt as per taste*

*Extra virgin olive oil*

*2 eggs, optional*

## STEPS FOR COOKING

1. Take a pan and heat butter
2. Sauté all vegetables and boil them for 5 – 7 minutes
3. Drain the extra water, which can be used for soups
4. Whip cream in a separate bowl and add beaten eggs (if required) with the cream
5. Pour the cream (with eggs) into the cooked vegetables
6. Add cheese and cook/bake for about 30 minutes, till it sets
7. Allow it to cool, cut, and serve

## INGREDIENTS

*2 cup sour cream*
*½ cup cheddar cheese*

## STEPS FOR COOKING

# Mexican Cauliflower Rice

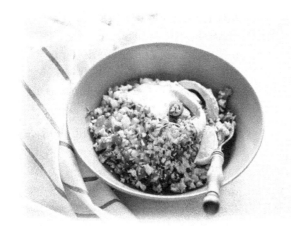

Time required:
25 minutes

Servings: 04

## INGREDIENTS

*1 head cauliflower, riced*

*1 tbsp olive oil*

*1 medium white onion, finely diced*

*2 cloves garlic, minced*

*1 jalapeno, seeded and minced*

*3 tbsp tomato paste*

*1 tsp sea salt*

*1 tsp cumin*

*1/2 tsp paprika*

*3 tbsp fresh chopped cilantro*

*1 tbsp lime juice*

## STEPS FOR COOKING

1. Rice the cauliflower. Slice the florets from the head of the cauliflower. Fit a food processor with the s-blade. Place half the florets into the bowl of the food processor and pulse until riced, scraping down the sides once halfway through to catch any larger pieces. Scrape out the riced cauliflower and repeat with the remaining florets.

2. Heat a skillet over medium-high heat. Add the oil and heat until it shimmers. Add the onion and saute until soft and translucent, stirring occasionally, 5-6 minutes.

3. Add the garlic and jalapeno and saute until fragrant, 1-2 minutes. Add the tomato paste, salt, cumin, and paprika and stir into the vegetables.

## INGREDIENTS

*½ cup feta cheese (tofu can be used instead)*

## STEPS FOR COOKING

4. Add the cauliflower rice and stir continuously until all ingredients are incorporated. Continue sautéing, stirring occasionally, until the cauliflower releases its liquid and is dry and fluffy.

5. Remove the Mexican cauliflower rice from heat. Stir in the cilantro and lime juice. Serve immediately.

# Chocolate Mug Cake

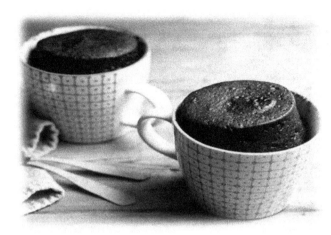

Time required:
5 minutes

Servings: 01

## INGREDIENTS

2 1/2 tbsp all-purpose flour

2 1/2 tbsp sugar

1 tbsp unsweetened cocoa powder

1/4 tsp baking powder

Pinch of salt

2 tbsp milk

1 tsp oil (canola, veg, sunflower)

1 small egg*

2 tbsp chocolate chips

## STEPS FOR COOKING

1.  With a fork, combine the flour, sugar, cocoa powder, baking powder, and salt in a microwave-safe mug.

2.  Whisk together the milk, grease, egg, and chocolate chips until a smooth cake batter forms.

3.  Microwave the cake for 45 seconds to 1 minute, or until it has risen and feels solid to the touch. take caution not to overcook the cake, or it will get complicated. (the timing depends on your microwave.)

4.  Until baked, serve with a dollop of fudge frosting, a dollop of whipped cream or ice cream, and some sprinkles.

# Leeks and Walnuts

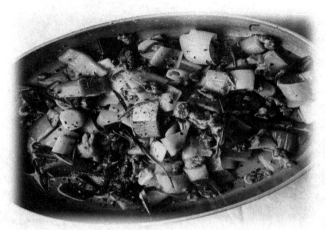

Time required:
4 hours

Servings: 06

| INGREDIENTS | STEPS FOR COOKING |
|---|---|

*1 tablespoon olive oil*

*4 leeks, roughly sliced*

*½ teaspoon dried thyme*

*½ cup chopped walnuts*

*2 tablespoons chicken stock*

*¼ cup chopped parsley*

1. Grease the slow cooker with the oil, add all the ingredients, cover, and cook on low for 4 hours.

# Rosemary Brussels Sprout

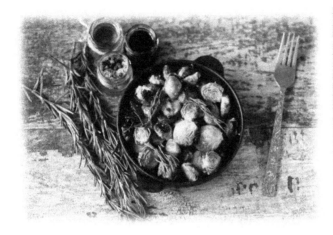

Time required:
5 hours

Servings: 06

## INGREDIENTS

*1 cup red onion, chopped*

*2 pounds Brussels sprout, halved*

*A pinch of salt and black pepper*

*½ cup vegetable stock*

*1 tablespoon coconut oil, melted*

*1 tablespoon chopped rosemary*

## STEPS FOR COOKING

1. In your slow cooker, combine all the ingredients, cover, and cook on low for 5 hours.

# Standard Greek Salad

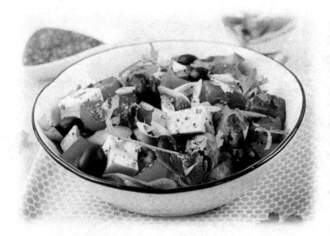

Time required:
15 minutes

Servings: 04

## INGREDIENTS

1 large tomato, cut
into cubes

1 cucumber, sliced
into half-moons

1/3 cup kalamata
olives, halved

1/2 white onion,
sliced

3/4 cup feta,
crumbled

2 tablespoon red
wine vinegar

2 tablespoon lemon
juice

1 teaspoon oregano,
dried

Salt and pepper to
taste

## STEPS FOR COOKING

1. In a separate bowl, combine the
   tomatoes, cucumbers, olives, and
   onion. Stir and top the mix with feta.

2. In another bowl, stir together the
   lemon juice, vinegar, oregano, salt,
   pepper, and olive oil. Gently whisk.

3. Sprinkle the salad with the dressing.

## INGREDIENTS

*1/4 cup extra-virgin olive oil*

## STEPS FOR COOKING

# Tofu Spinach Sauté

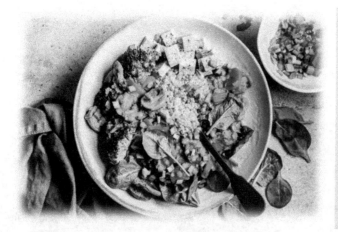

Time required:
25 minutes

---

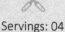

Servings: 04

## INGREDIENTS

1/4 cup onion,
chopped

1/4 cup button
mushrooms,
chopped

8 ounces tofu,
pressed and
chopped

3 teaspoons
nutritional yeast

1 teaspoon liquid
aminos

4 cups baby spinach

4 grape tomatoes,
chopped

Cooking spray

## STEPS FOR COOKING

1. Sauté mushrooms and onion with oil in a skillet for 3 minutes.

2. Stir in tofu and sauté for 3 minutes.

3. Add liquid aminos and yeast then mix well.

4. Stir in tomatoes and spinach then sauté for 4 minutes.

5. Serve warm.

# Chicken Zucchini

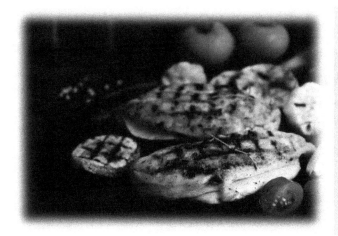

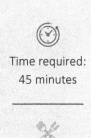

Time required:
45 minutes

Servings: 04

## INGREDIENTS

4 pieces of chicken breast

1 cup Zucchini, chopped

2 tablespoons shredded cheese

1 raw onion, chopped

Salt, to taste

Black pepper, to taste

Oregano, to taste

## STEPS FOR COOKING

1. At 450 degrees F, preheat your oven.
2. Place the chicken breast in a baking pan and drizzle oregano, black pepper and salt on top.
3. Drizzle cheese on top and cover the chicken with zucchini slices.
4. Bake this chicken for 30 minutes in the oven.
5. Serve warm.

# Sardine Fish Cakes

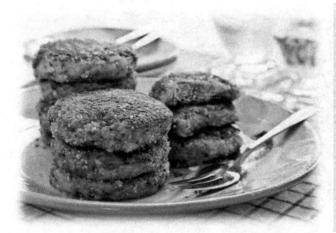

Time required:
25 minutes

Servings: 04

## INGREDIENTS

11 oz. sardines, canned, drained

1/3 cup shallot, chopped

1 teaspoon chili flakes

½ teaspoon salt

2 tablespoon wheat flour, whole grain

1 egg, beaten

1 tablespoon chives, chopped

1 teaspoon butter

## STEPS FOR COOKING

1. Put the butter in your skillet and dissolve it. Add shallot and cook it until translucent. After this, transfer the shallot to the mixing bowl.

2. Add sardines, chili flakes, salt, flour, egg, chives, and mix up until smooth with the fork's help. Make the medium size cakes and place them in the skillet. Add olive oil.

3. Roast the fish cakes for 3 minutes from each side over medium heat. Dry the cooked fish cakes with a paper towel if needed and transfer to the serving plates.

# Beef & Mushroom Chili

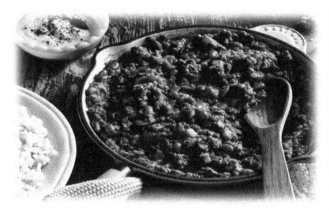

Time required:
3 hours

Servings: 08

## INGREDIENTS

*2 pounds grass-fed ground beef*

*1 yellow onion*

*1/2 cup green bell pepper*

*1/2 cup carrot*

*4 ounces mushrooms*

*2 garlic cloves*

*1 can sugar-free tomato paste*

*2 tablespoons red chili powder*

*1 tablespoon ground cumin*

*1 teaspoon ground cinnamon*

*1 teaspoon red pepper flakes*

## STEPS FOR COOKING

1. Cook the beef within 8–10 minutes. Stir in the remaining ingredients except for sour cream and boil. Cook on low, covered, within 3 hours.

2. Top with sour cream and serve.

## INGREDIENTS

*1/2 teaspoon ground allspice*

*Salt to taste*

*Ground black pepper to taste*

*4 cups of water*

*1/2 cup sour cream*

## STEPS FOR COOKING

# Spanish Cod in Sauce

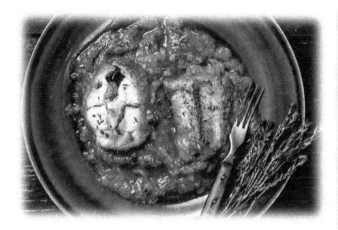

Time required:
20 minutes

Servings: 02

## INGREDIENTS

*1 teaspoon tomato paste*

*1 teaspoon garlic, diced*

*1 white onion, sliced*

*1 jalapeno pepper, chopped*

*1/3 cup chicken stock*

*7 oz. Spanish cod fillet*

*1 teaspoon paprika*

*1 teaspoon salt*

## STEPS FOR COOKING

1. Pour chicken stock into the saucepan. Add tomato paste and mix up the liquid until homogenous. Add garlic, onion, jalapeno pepper, paprika, and salt.

2. Bring the liquid to boil and then simmer it. Chop the cod fillet and add it to the tomato liquid. Simmer the fish for 10 minutes over low heat. Serve the fish in the bowls with tomato sauce.

# Pesto Cream Veggie Dip

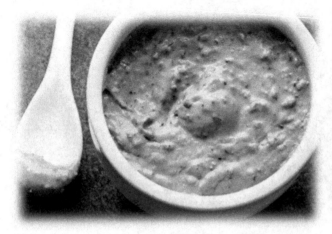

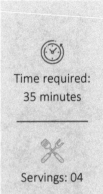

Time required:
35 minutes

Servings: 04

## INGREDIENTS

*100g (3½oz) cream cheese*
*200g (7oz) basil pesto*
*2 tablespoons parmesan cheese*
*100g (3½oz) sour cream*

## STEPS FOR COOKING

1. Place cream cheese, sour cream, pesto, and parmesan cheese in a bowl and stir well.
2. Stir until chill and creamy.
3. Ready to serve.

# Eggs Souffle

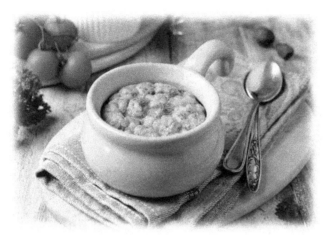

Time required:
25 minutes

Servings: 02

## INGREDIENTS

*3 egg yolks and
whites separately
2 tablespoons milk
2 tablespoons
gluten-free flour
Garlic salt, pepper,
100 g English bacon*

## STEPS FOR COOKING

1. Preheat the oven to 190 degrees C.
2. Beat the yolks with milk and flour,
   Season with garlic salt and pepper.
3. Whisk the egg whites into the solid
   snow, lightly add to the base.

# Chicken and Broccoli Casserole

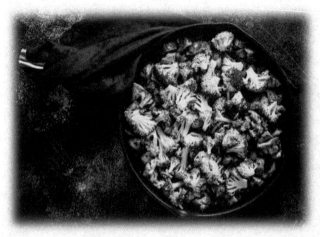

Time required:
25 minutes

Servings: 02

## INGREDIENTS

*1 1/2 lbs chicken breast without bone, cut into cubes*

*1/4 tsp every salt and pepper*

*10 oz frozen broccoli florets*

*8 oz fat-free cream of celery soup*

*1/4 cup of unsweet, unflavored almond milk*

*1/2 cup of shredded reduced fat cheddar cheese*

## STEPS FOR COOKING

1. Preheat the oven to 375 degrees Fahrenheit. Use a 13x9 baking dish with cooking spray. Place the chicken in the baking dish and season it with salt and pepper.

2. Bake for 15 minutes, or thoroughly cooked. Thaw and drink the broccoli while the chicken is frying.

3. Add the broccoli mixture to the casserole dish and spread the chicken mixture evenly around the plate with a rubber spatula. Mix all in thoroughly.

4. Add the broccoli mixture to the casserole dish and spread the chicken mixture evenly around the plate with a rubber spatula. Then using a fork, thinly distribute the cheese on top.

5. Bake until the sides begin to bubble and the top starts to brown slightly.

# Strawberry Salad with Orange Balsamic Dressing

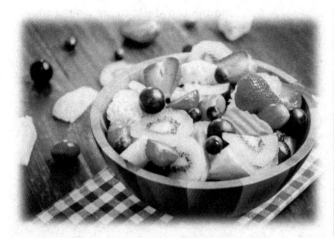

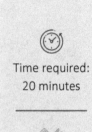

Time required:
20 minutes

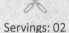

Servings: 02

| INGREDIENTS | STEPS FOR COOKING |
|---|---|
| *60 g of banana*<br>*100 g strawberries (frozen)*<br>*100 g raspberries (frozen)*<br>*300 ml soy milk*<br>*1 tbsp maple syrup*<br>*1 teaspoon lime juice*<br>*Some fresh lemon balm*<br>*A handful of Fresh raspberries* | 1. Peel the banana and put it in the blender with the frozen strawberries and raspberries and mix briefly to a puree.<br>2. Then add the soy milk, maple syrup and 1 teaspoon lime juice and mix again briefly.<br>3. Divide the shake between two glasses, decorate with the fresh raspberries and lemon balm and serve. |

# Potato Dumplings

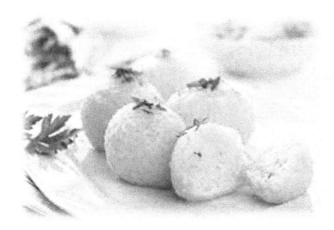

Time required:
35 minutes

Servings: 04

## INGREDIENTS

*900 g potatoes*

*15 g fresh, flat-leaf parsley*

*6 teaspoons of olive oil*

*1 teaspoon herbal salt*

*Some ground nutmeg*

*Slightly ground white pepper*

*A steamer is also required.*

## STEPS FOR COOKING

1. First, wash the potatoes and cut them into small pieces. Then put the potatoes in a steamer and steam until soft for about 15 minutes.

2. Meanwhile, wash the parsley, pat dry and pluck the leaves from the stems.

3. Save a few for decoration later and finely chop the rest.

4. Now take the potatoes out of the steamer and mash them with a fork. Then add the olive oil, the grated nutmeg, the chopped parsley, the herb salt and the pepper and mix well.

5. Now shape the mixture into dumplings using two tablespoons, arrange on four plates and serve garnished with parsley.

# Konjac Pasta

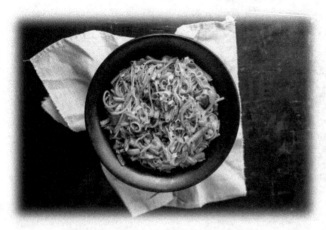

Time required:
35 minutes

Servings: 04

## INGREDIENTS

500 g konjac
noodles

900 g paprika

100 g green olives

40 g capers

2 cloves of garlic

4 teaspoons of olive
oil

Some fresh oregano

Some fresh parsley

salt

pepper

## STEPS FOR COOKING

1. First, rinse the pasta thoroughly until it is odorless. Then wash the oregano and parsley, pat dry and finely chop. Then wash the peppers and cut in half. Also, pit and halve the olives. Finally, finely chop the capers.

2. Set the oven to 180 ° C fan oven and place the peppers on a wire shelf. Let cook on the middle shelf for about 15 minutes. Then put it in a freezer bag and allow it to evaporate so that the shell begins to loosen easily. Now the skin can be easily peeled off. Now halve the peppers, remove the seeds and puree in a blender to a fine cream.

3. Then put the olive oil in a saucepan, heat it and sweat the garlic in it. Now pour on the paprika cream, add the

| INGREDIENTS | STEPS FOR COOKING |
|---|---|
| | chopped capers and olives and stir well. |
| | 4. Finally, add the konjak noodles and let them steep for a few minutes. Finally season with salt and pepper, top with the parsley and oregano and serve. |

# Light Tomato Soup

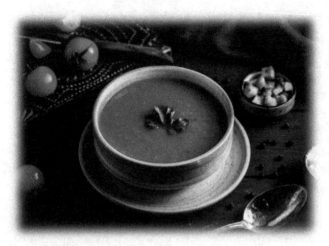

Time required:
35 minutes

Servings: 02

## INGREDIENTS

*250 g tomatoes*

*30 g carrots*

*15 g celery*

*25 g leek*

*2 teaspoons of oatmeal*

*0.5 tsp vegetable broth*

*0.5 tsp dried oregano*

*1 small pinch of salt*

*1 small Pinch of nutmeg*

## STEPS FOR COOKING

1. First, wash the tomatoes thoroughly, remove the stalks and cut into pieces. Then wash and finely dice the celery and leek. Now wash the carrots, peel them and also cut them into small cubes.

2. Bring 1 liter of water to the boil in a large saucepan, add the vegetable stock and add the vegetables. Simmer gently over low heat for about 15 minutes until everything is soft.

3. Now strain the soup through a sieve and season with salt, nutmeg and oregano. Put the tomato soup in two soup cups, sprinkle with the oatmeal and serve.

# Nutmeg Pumpkin Soup

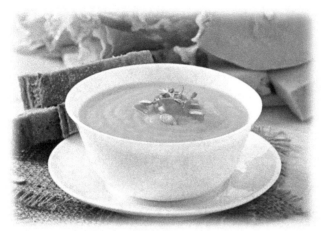

Time required:
35 minutes

Servings: 04

## INGREDIENTS

1 tablespoon of butter

1 onion, diced

1(16-ounces) can of pumpkin puree

1/3 cups of vegetable broth

1/2 tablespoon of nutmeg

1/2 tablespoon of sugar

Salt, to taste

Pepper, to taste

3 cups of soymilk or any milk as a substitute

## STEPS FOR COOKING

1. Using a large saucepan, add onion to margarine and cook it between 3 and 5 minutes until the onion is clear.

2. Add pumpkin puree, vegetable broth, sugar, pepper, and other ingredients and stir to combine.

3. Cook in medium heat for between 10 and fifteen minutes.

4. Before serving the soup, taste and add more spices, pepper, and salt if necessary.

5. Serve soup and enjoy it!

# Baked Rice Pan with Vegetables

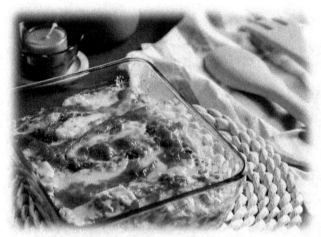

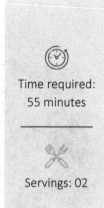

Time required:
55 minutes

_____

Servings: 02

| INGREDIENTS | STEPS FOR COOKING |
|---|---|

*100 g kohlrabi*

*1 red pepper*

*2 carrots*

*10 cherry tomatoes*

*2 small onions*

*1 clove of garlic*

*2 tbsp olive oil*

*130 g paella rice*

*1 teaspoon hot
paprika powder*

*400 ml vegetable
stock*

*½ lemon salt pepper*

*100 g low-fat yogurt*

*2 spring onions*

1. Preheat the oven to 180 ° C.
2. Wash the kohlrabi. Clean and peel it. Peel the carrots and onions and cut them into cubes. Peel and chop the garlic. Wash the pepper. Then cut them into four pieces and core them. Roughly dice them. Wash the cherry tomatoes.
3. Heat the olive oil in a pan. Add the onions and garlic and sauté them until they turn translucent. Add the kohlrabi, carrots and bell peppers and steam them for 2 minutes.
4. Add the rice and steam it briefly. Pour the broth over it and bring it to a boil. Stir and season everything with salt and pepper.

5. Put the rice pan in the oven and bake it on the bottom rack. After 10 minutes, take them out briefly and place the cherry tomatoes on top. Then bake them for another 10 minutes and take them out of the oven.

6. Meanwhile, squeeze out the lemon and measure out a teaspoon of lemon juice. Mix it with the yogurt and paprika powder.

7. Wash and clean the spring onions. Cut them into fine rings and sprinkle them over the vegetable and rice pan. Serve them with the paprika yogurt.

# Creamy Mushrooms with Potatoes

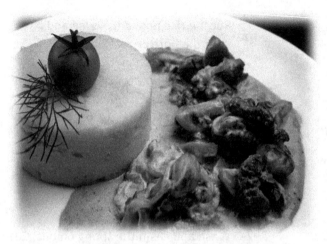

Time required:
30 minutes

Servings: 01

## INGREDIENTS

150 g potatoes

200 g mushrooms

1 shallot

1 stalk of tarragon

2 tbsp olive oil

80 ml vegetable stock

80 g sour cream

80 g romaine lettuce

salt

pepper

## STEPS FOR COOKING

1.  Peel the potatoes and wash them, cut them into small cubes. Clean the mushrooms and roughly dice them.

2.  Clean the shallot and dice it very finely. Wash the tarragon and shake it dry. Pluck the leaves off and cut it.

3.  In a pan heat 1 tablespoon of olive oil. Fry the potatoes for 10 minutes, turning them, and salt them.

4.  Then, heat the remaining olive oil in a second pan. Add the shallot and cook it. Add the mushrooms and fry them until the liquid has evaporated completely. Pour the vegetable stock over it. Season the vegetables with salt and pepper and let them simmer for 4-5 minutes. Add the sour cream and tarragon and stir everything well.

| INGREDIENTS | STEPS FOR COOKING |
|---|---|

5. Brush and wash the lettuce. Shake it dry and cut it into strips. Lift it under the mushrooms and serve it with the potatoes.

# Grilled Steak

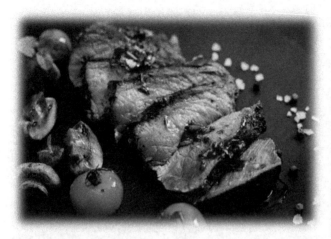

Time required:
15 minutes

Servings: 06

## INGREDIENTS

*1 teaspoon lemon zest*

*1 garlic clove*

*1 tablespoon red chili powder*

*1 tablespoon paprika*

*1 tablespoon ground coffee*

*Salt to taste*

*Ground black pepper to taste*

*2 grass-fed skirt steaks*

## STEPS FOR COOKING

1. Mix all the ingredients except steaks. Marinate the steaks and keep them aside within 30–40 minutes.

2. Grill the steaks within 5–6 minutes per side. Remove and then cool before slicing. Serve.

# Baked Pears with Yogurt and Cinnamon

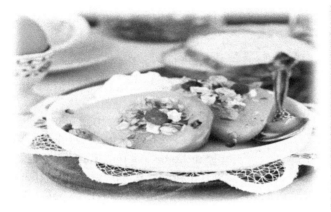

Time required:
35 minutes

Servings: 02

## INGREDIENTS

*20 g walnut kernels*

*2 small firm pears*

*½ lime*

*2 teaspoons maple syrup*

*100 g yogurt*

*ground cinnamon*

## STEPS FOR COOKING

1. Preheat the oven to 200 ° C.

2. Heat a pan over medium heat. Chop the walnuts and roast them until they have turned golden brown. Put them aside.

3. Wash and dry the pears.

4. Cut 2 sheets of parchment paper to about 25x30 cm. Place them side by side on a baking sheet.

5. Squeeze out the lime. Put the lime juice in a bowl along with 1 teaspoon maple syrup. Add the walnuts and stir all the ingredients.

6. Place two halves of pear in the middle of the baking paper and drizzle the walnut-syrup mixture over them.

7. Tie the sheets of parchment paper together at both ends with twine like candy. Seal them well.

| INGREDIENTS | STEPS FOR COOKING |
|---|---|

**STEPS FOR COOKING**

8. Bake the pears on the middle rack for 10 minutes.

9. Meanwhile, put the yogurt and cinnamon in a small bowl and stir the ingredients well.

10. Take the pears out of the oven and place them on a plate. Carefully unfold the baking paper and drizzle the remaining maple syrup over the pears. Serve them with the yogurt.

11. Add the orange peel and salt. Put the cream in a container. Put them in the freezer for at least 3 hours.

# Berry Parfait

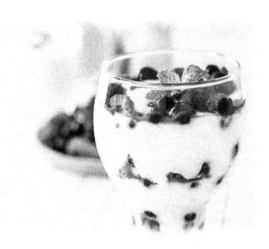

Time required:
25 minutes

Servings: 04

| INGREDIENTS | STEPS FOR COOKING |
|---|---|

*14 oz. / 400 g mixed berries*

*1 tsp. honey*

*3.5 oz. / 100 g Greek yogurt*

*7 oz. / 200 g almond butter*

*7 oz. / 200 g mixed nuts*

1. Combine the Greek yogurt, butter, and honey until it's smooth.
2. Put in a layer of berries and a layer of the mixture in a glass until it's full.
3. Serve instantly with sprinkled nuts.

# Turmeric-Almond Smoothie

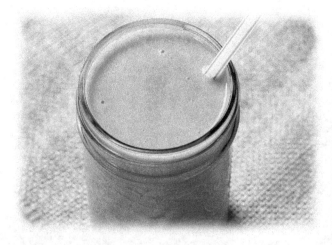

Time required:
10 minutes

Servings: 02

## INGREDIENTS

*1 pear, cored and
quartered cups baby
spinach*

*¼ avocado*

*1 cup silken tofu*

*1 teaspoon ground
turmeric or 1 thin
slice of peeled
turmeric root*

*½ cup unsweetened
almond milk*

*2 tablespoons honey
(optional)*

*1 cup ice*

## STEPS FOR COOKING

1. Combine in a blender, all the
   ingredients and blend until smooth.
   Divide between two glasses and serve.

2. Substitution tip: if pears aren't in
   season, you can substitute an apple
   for similar flavor and nutritional
   rewards.

# Rosemary Lemon Iced Tea

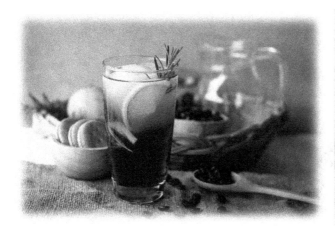

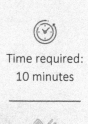

Time required:
10 minutes

Servings: 02

## INGREDIENTS

½ cup of sugar

4 cups of water

One sprig of
rosemary

2 lemons

4 tea bags

## STEPS FOR COOKING

1. Peel the lemons but don't take too much of the white part into the peels because it will make the tea bitter.

2. In a small-sized pot, add water, lemon peels, and sugar. Boil.

3. Remove the pot and add the tea bags and the rosemary sprig. Keep the lid on and leave the pot aside for five minutes.

4. Strain the tea and remove the tea bags. Take the peeled lemons, juice them, and add the juice into the tea. Serve chilled over ice.

# Blueberry Muffins

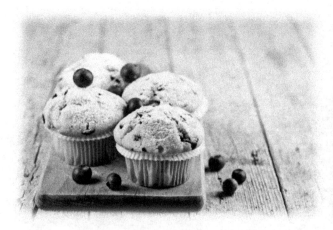

Time required:
45 minutes

---

Servings: 08

## INGREDIENTS

2½ cups almond flour

1 tablespoon coconut flour

½ tsp baking soda

3 tablespoons ground cinnamon, divided

Salt, to taste

2 organic eggs

¼ cup coconut milk

¼ cup coconut oil

¼ cup maple syrup

1 tablespoon organic vanilla flavor

1 cup fresh blueberries

## STEPS FOR COOKING

1. Preheat the oven to 350 degrees F. Grease 10 cups of a large muffin tin.

2. In a big bowl, mix together flours, baking soda, 2 tablespoons of cinnamon and salt.

3. In another bowl, add eggs, milk, oil, maple syrup and vanilla and beat till well combined.

4. Add egg mixture into flour mixture and mix till well combined.

5. Fold in blueberries.

6. Place a combination into prepared muffin cups evenly.

7. Sprinkle with cinnamon evenly.

8. Bake for approximately 22-25 minutes or till a toothpick inserted within the center is released clean.

# Chocolate Mug Cake

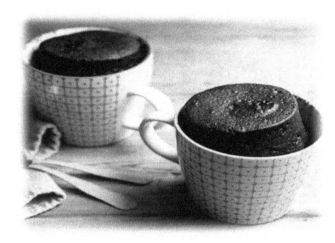

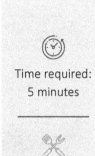

Time required:
5 minutes

Servings: 01

## INGREDIENTS

*2 1/2 tbsp all-purpose flour*

*2 1/2 tbsp sugar*

*1 tbsp unsweetened cocoa powder*

*1/4 tsp baking powder*

*Pinch of salt*

*2 tbsp milk*

*1 tsp oil (canola, veg, sunflower)*

*1 small egg\**

*2 tbsp chocolate chips*

## STEPS FOR COOKING

1. With a fork, combine the flour, sugar, cocoa powder, baking powder, and salt in a microwave-safe mug.

2. Whisk together the milk, grease, egg, and chocolate chips until a smooth cake batter forms.

3. Microwave the cake for 45 seconds to 1 minute, or until it has risen and feels solid to the touch. take caution not to overcook the cake, or it will get complicated. (the timing depends on your microwave.)

4. Until baked, serve with a dollop of fudge frosting, a dollop of whipped cream or ice cream, and some sprinkles.

# Banana Bars

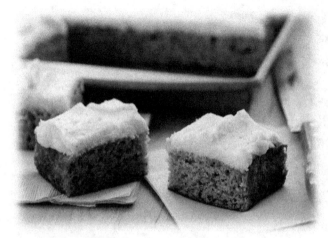

Time required:
60 minutes

—

Servings: 04

## INGREDIENTS

*½ cup Coconut Milk*

*½ cup Melted Butter*

*1 cup Chocolate Chips*

*1 tsp. Baking Soda*

*1 tsp. Pure Vanilla Extract*

*1/4 tbsp. Cinnamon*

*1 cup Brown Sugar*

*2 cup Whole Wheat Flour*

*2 eggs*

*1 cup Ripe Mashed Banana*

*Salt*

## STEPS FOR COOKING

1. Preheat your oven to 170 ºC.
2. Mix all together the ingredients to make the batter.
3. Put the batter in a wide tray and bake for about twenty minutes at 170 ºC.
4. Serve with liquid chocolate or fruits.

# Orange Avocado Smoothie

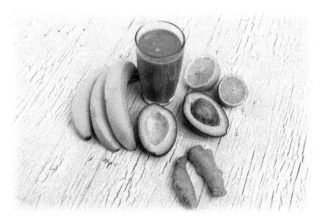

Time required:
15 minutes

Servings: 02

| INGREDIENTS | STEPS FOR COOKING |
|---|---|
| *2 handfuls of green leafy vegetables* <br> *1 cup of water* <br> *6 ice cubes* <br> *3 oranges, juice* <br> *½ avocado* | 1. Wash, drain and roughly chop the leafy vegetables. Halve the avocado and cut the pulp into small pieces. <br><br> 2. Put all ingredients in a blender and puree very finely. |

# Walnut Banana Muffin

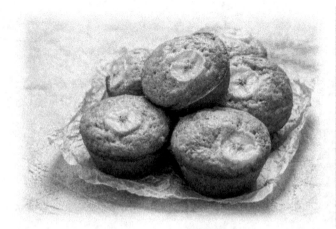

Time required:
35 minutes

Servings: 02

## INGREDIENTS

*3 cups spelt-flour*

*2 cups walnut milk*

*3 ripe bananas, mashed + 1 into chunks*

*1 cup date sugar*

*1 tbsp lime juice*

*½ cup grapeseed oil*

*1 cup walnuts, chopped*

*1 pinch teaspoon sea salt*

## STEPS FOR COOKING

1. Heat your oven to 400F.
2. Mix spelt salt and date sugar, add mashed bananas, oil, lime juice, and mix well.
3. Add walnut milk and stir well. Add walnut chunks and mix.
4. Divide the batter into each muffin cup and cook 25 minutes until golden brown.

# Chocolate Balls

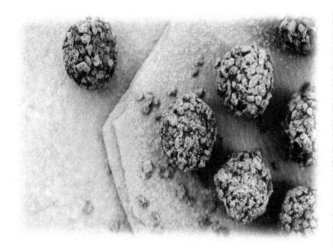

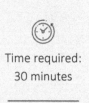

Time required:
30 minutes

Servings: 10

## INGREDIENTS

*1 cup of rolled oats*

*½ cup of natural peanut butter*

*⅓ cup of honey*

*¼ cup of chopped dark chocolate*

*2 tbsp flax seeds*

*2 tbsp chia seeds*

*1 tbsp chocolate-flavored protein powder, or as need*

## STEPS FOR COOKING

1. In a mixing cup, combine rice, peanut butter, sugar, cocoa, flax seeds, chia seeds, and protein powder until uniformly mixed. Refrigerate for 30 minutes after wrapping the bowl in plastic wrap.

2. Make balls out of the chilled mixture. Keep chilled until ready to serve.

CPSIA information can be obtained
at www.ICGtesting.com
Printed in the USA
BVHW091928230621
610293BV00008B/1194